I0411412

10 REASONS TO NOT IGNORE

REFLUX OR HEARTBURN

CLIFF THOMAS, MD

Dedicated

To My Uncle,
~ Clyde Thomas, MD ~

Contents

Introduction 7

GERD: The Burning Truth 11

    GERD: A Basic Understanding 12

    The Results of GERD 13

    Other Facts About GERD 14

    GERD: The Role of the Hiatal Hernia 14

    Getting Treatment 15

10 Reasons To Not Ignore Reflux or Heartburn 17

    1: Heartburn 18

    2: Esophagitis 18

    3: Esophageal Stricture 19

    4: Throat and Voice Problems 19

    5: Breathing Problems 20

    6: Tooth Decay 21

    7: Chronic Cough 21

    8: Sleep Problems 22

    9: Barrett's Esophagus 23

    10: Esophageal Cancer 24

    Why Is Cancer Of The Esophagus On The Rise? 25

7 Conditions That Mimic GERD **29**

   1: Stomach Ulcers and Gastritis... 30

   2: Heart Disease 30

   3: Gallbladder Disease.. 31

   4: Pleuritis or Costochondritis... 31

   5: Achalasia... 32

   6: Eosinophilic Esophagitis 33

   7: Functional Heartburn... 33

Diagnostic Process..**35**

   The Consultation and EGD.. 36

   Endoscopy 36

   Biopsies 37

   Barium X-ray 37

   Impedence 37

   Manometry... 38

   PH Testing.. 38

Common Problems Resulting From GERD Medication.................... **41**

   Prilosec... 42

   Nexium 42

   Prevacid 43

   Aciphex 44

   Dexilant.. 44

   Tagamet.. 45

   Pepcid... 46

   Gaviscon 46

Surgery…What Are Your Options? **47**

   Nissen Fundoplication.. 49

   TIF or Transoral Incisionless Fundoplication 51

   Stretta Procedure 52

Living Without GERD: Choosing a Life You Love **53**

   The Good News! 54

   Great Possibilities 54

   Regain Your Freedom 55

Final Words..**55**

About the Author..**57**

Introduction

You or someone you know has bad acid reflux. It is that common and that under treated. I wrote this book to hopefully expand everyday understanding of GERD and the problems it is causing.

I have a passion for treating patients with reflux. I have had the amazing experience of doing so for twenty-five years. It is fun to see patients back after surgery and have them report similar to what Carol said, "*Reflux surgery is one of the three best things I have done in life - getting married, having kids, and having reflux surgery.*"

Not everyone with reflux needs surgery, but those are the most rewarding to treat because reflux symptoms are dramatically interfering with their life.

For twenty-five years I have had patients come to my office and later ask after having surgery, "*Why didn't my doctor send me or recommend this to me sooner*".

I will explain why, but first I want explain why there is a difference in opinion and skewed results.

The difference in opinion comes from a differing approach to treating a medical problem. We have lived many decades thinking we can add chemistry of some sort to our bodies without significant consequences. We now have our food laced with all kinds of chemicals and I personally think that is a major cause of why we seem to be getting less healthy despite all the new medical breakthroughs. We have been living in an age where we thought there was a pill for every problem no matter how simple. However, times are changing and people are realizing that's not good. People are leaning towards organic foods hoping they are laced with fewer chemicals.

People are realizing that taking antibiotics for every little thing messes up their gut flora and that makes them less healthy. Anti-inflammatory drugs do help with the suffering of daily aches and pains, but consequently our gut has impaired absorption of nutrients. These are just two examples of drugs that make the gut less able to do its job as designed. It is less able to digest and absorb the important nutrients that power our bodies.

Now, we are finding that the drugs used to treat reflux may cause problems with weakening of bones as well as some drug interactions. Medical doctors like to treat with medicines. Surgical doctors like to treat with surgery. I personally do both.

The medicines are safe particularly compared to other medications. But they do not fix the underlying problem, which is a mechanical problem, not a chemistry problem. Many people have thought they had an acid problem with too much acid, but that's not true. Rarely does someone have too much acid. The acid is just in a place where it does not belong, the esophagus, and that causes symptoms and damage.

The mechanical problem is a broken one -way valve. When we eat, our food goes from our mouth into a tube called the esophagus. The muscles in the esophagus squeeze first at the top, then the middle, and then the end, pushing the food out of the esophagus and into the stomach. The esophagus has a non-acid environment. The stomach has many digestive chemicals that are caustic or can burn if not in the stomach. They are acid, bile, and enzymes.

There is a one-way valve at the end of the esophagus that should allow food to pass from the esophagus to the stomach, but not come back up. When that valve is broken, then caustic stomach juices can go up into the esophagus where they do not belong and cause damage, pain, and cancer. It is like any broken valve we might encounter in daily life, like our toilets. When the valve in our toilet is broken, it leaks water. You can live with it leaking if you can stand the sound and pay the water bill, but the only way to fix it is to change to a new working one-way valve.

Some surgeons simply do not know how to do the surgery correctly and do not have good results. Surgeons that are passionate about the esophagus and perform the surgeries routinely, like weekly, have excellent long-term results. Most doctors have not had the experience of referring to an experienced surgeon and therefore are unaware of the excellent results. However, it is well documented in study after study that surgeons who perform reflux surgery routinely have a 95% or more, success rate.

So for years this has been the typical scenario. A patient complains of reflux symptoms to their doctor and he refers them to a gastroenterologist who can diagnose and treat reflux with medicine, but cannot do surgery and often does not know a good surgeon to refer to. So they do a procedure called endoscopy where the gastroenterologist looks into the esophagus and stomach with a scope. The gastroenterologist then diagnoses GERD and writes a prescription and that is the end of it. Some patients do very well on the medicine, but many despite some improvement still have significant symptoms yet nothing more is suggested. Referral to a surgeon is rarely discussed.

I believe in a balance approach.

Times are changing. The number of people now reporting reflux symptoms and being diagnosed with GERD is skyrocketing.

We don't know why. It probably is a combination of medications, food additives, and over eating.

There is now a very important reason to pay more attention to GERD. The number of new cases of esophageal cancer is also skyrocketing and there is compelling evidence it is related to GERD. Treatment of GERD with medicine does not seem to decrease this risk. We believe surgical treatment where the one-way valve is re-built does decrease this risk. It will take many years to prove, but the work by some pathologist makes this seem true.

So it is time we get busy and increase our attention to reflux. Read and pay attention to the 10 reasons to not ignore reflux and heartburn.

GERD: The Burning Truth

Have you ever experienced a really bad case of heartburn? Then you know just how painful and uncomfortable it can be. It begins as a burning sensation in your chest, which tends to creep up into your throat. My patients say that heartburn feels like burning juices flowing back up their throats.

When a person refluxes, their stomach acids flow back into their esophagus, causing that scratchy, burning feeling during and after the experience. Some people experience more severe effects when they reflux, which causes restricted breathing, and makes them feel like they're having a full blown heart attack!

For those of you who suffer with the pain of heartburn often, there is little doubt as to how disruptive and damaging this condition can be. It is normal for someone to get heartburn once a month or so, but when it happens frequently, that is when the trouble strikes. If you have heartburn several times a month, then you need to start taking it seriously. At this point, it is wise to consult your doctor about your condition.

Did you know that...?

Heartburn is one of the most
common symptoms of GERD

Heartburn can result in many other health issues, and there are a few of these that can only be caught if your cells are studied directly under a microscope, and we do that by performing a procedure called endoscopy.

To date, there are about 19 million people that suffer with severe heartburn, and are diagnosed with GERD, or Gastro esophageal Reflux Disease. The terms 'heartburn' and 'acid reflux' are heard all the time, but few people are familiar with GERD. It is important to understand what is going on inside your body!

GERD: A Basic Understanding

GERD is essentially a reflux disease. When you eat, the food that you swallow should move from the back of your tongue, to your esophagus and into your stomach. At the end of your esophagus, and the beginning of your stomach – sits the lower esophagus sphincter, or the one-way valve we've been speaking about. Food is only supposed to flow one way.

Food and juices should enter your stomach, and not climb back up into your esophagus. But, when you have a valve problem the food shoots up into your esophagus again, which causes pain in the nerve pathways and damage to your throat. That is why GERD can be defined as a digestive condition that causes dysfunction in your lower esophageal sphincter.

GERD can flare up for any number of reasons – including changes in diet or pregnancy. But, GERD is the stepping-stone to more severe health conditions, so it is dangerous to leave it untreated.

You can improve GERD by adjusting your diet, and making appropriate lifestyle changes – like reducing stress, or quitting smoking and drinking alcohol. People who are overweight and have been diagnosed with GERD often experience relief if they lose weight. Lifestyle changes are encouraged, but rarely followed. If one eats or drinks wine, tomato sauce, Mexican food, and the like, it causes heartburn repeatedly. They still keep eating it and I doubt a doctor telling them to stop eating it will work any better. The bottom line is that lifestyle changes do not fix the reflux problem and are rarely followed.

Did you know that…?
Lifestyle changes such as dietary changes
can often reduce GERD symptoms

The Results of GERD

As I mentioned before, GERD is a gateway condition, which can lead to many other health problems. This depends on the severity of the disease, and on how much damage has occurred to the LES (lower esophagus sphincter). The length of time a person has lived with untreated acid reflux, heartburn and GERD, is also a factor. There are a number of related problems a patient will experience, which exceeds the pain and discomfort of having GERD.

Over-the-counter medication is often the go-to solution for patients that suffer from GERD. If your symptoms get worse, or they occur more often, then it is time to talk to your doctor. This becomes even more important when the severity of your pain and discomfort from GERD increases. Do not leave it untreated!

Other Facts About GERD

The medical field is still learning about problems related to digestion and what triggers these conditions. One of the most common misconceptions about GERD is that it only flares up when you eat spicy foods.

While certain foods have been linked to heartburn and acid reflux, they are certainly not the cause. Foods like peppermint, chocolate and fried foods can also cause reflux, along with coffee and alcohol. All of these foods have been linked to increasing the chance of experiencing heartburn.

But it is not only food that can cause an increase in these symptoms. Straining or bending over can aggravate the symptoms. When GERD happens, people feel the need to lie down in order to control the pain. Lying down tends to make the problem worse. For these reasons, you need to steer clear of eating just before you go to bed, especially if you're prone to heartburn and indigestion.

GERD: The Role of the Hiatal Hernia

Research has indicated that a hiatal hernia can weaken the LES, which dramatically increases your chances of contracting GERD. A hiatal hernia happens when the upper part of your stomach pokes through a small opening in your diaphragm, or chest. Your diaphragm is the muscle that separates your chest from your abdomen. People that have a hiatal hernia, tend to experience a lot of problems with heartburn. This is because your hernia allows your stomach contents to reflux into your esophagus more easily.

A hiatal hernia is caused by weakening of the support structures around the esophagus. We do not know why this happens, but it does.

Just because you have a hiatal hernia doesn't mean you need surgery. But sometimes, if the hernia is very large it may be at risk of twisting and cutting off blood supply (paraesophageal hernia), or worsening the severity GERD and treatment will be necessary. In these cases, a surgeon will reduce the size of the hernia in surgery.

Did you know that…?
The intensity of the GERD symptoms does
not correlate with the severity of damage

Getting Treatment

It is important to understand that the degree that symptoms cause pain and discomfort does not tell us how much damage there may be to the esophagus. A person can have mild symptoms and severe damage, and a person can have severe symptoms and no tissue damage. Symptoms are a poor indicator of the severity of the disease. If a person has frequent symptoms, they need endoscopy and further evaluation.

If you suffer from heartburn on a daily or weekly basis, this is a clear warning sign that something is wrong. Even if you only experience it a few times a month, it is better to have it checked out by your doctor. Effective treatments are out there, so do not wait until it is too late to get the treatment that you need.

10 Reasons To Not Ignore Reflux or Heartburn

GERD is an extremely uncomfortable condition to live with, but that is not the only reason why seeking treatment is important. Many untreated diseases like GERD result in a host of additional health problems. GERD could even be a symptom of a much more serious disease.

If you've been diagnosed with GERD, then you need to talk to your doctor about getting better treatment, before these other health concerns creep up on you. It is also a good idea to ask your doctor if they could check if GERD isn't perhaps a side effect of a more serious, life threatening illness.

Do not panic just yet. Many diseases and conditions can be cured, but first they have to be found and treated.

1: Heartburn

GERD is the leading cause of repetitive heartburn, and can be heightened in pregnant women, or as a side effect of medications like Cialis and others, or even from taking supplements like vitamin C.

The severity of heartburn symptoms does not correlate with the severity of tissue damage from GERD. A person can have mild symptoms and no tissue damage and a person can have severe incapacitating symptoms and no tissue damage.

In general, everyone that experiences a mild or a severe case of heartburn on a daily or weekly basis, needs to see a doctor. Heartburn can become more intense over time, and can become more frequent – especially if you just ignore it. Medical stats have shown that 60 million Americans suffer with heartburn or acid reflux disease. For every ten people, one of them deals with it daily, and 20% of them have weekly heartburn troubles.

2: Esophagitis

Esophagitis is the name given to damaged esophageal tissue. The diagnosis varies in intensity – from looking red and inflamed, to more severe versions. What you need to understand here, is that the visible appearance of your esophagus might not always indicate the true damage that it has experienced.

When you look under a microscope, the damage to your esophagus can become clearer, as more insight is given to the extent of your condition. In very severe cases, the esophagus has suffered so much damage that scarring and erosion has taken place, which means that it is not functioning properly, and is not sealing the pathway between your throat and stomach.

A crucial step is deciding that you need to have an endoscopy, so that you can match your symptoms to the damage that has been done.

Honestly, you cannot tell exactly how much damage has really been done, just by the symptoms you are having.

3: Esophageal Stricture

An esophageal stricture is a narrowing of the esophagus that leads to it tightening, which prevents you from swallowing properly. Food gets stuck on the way down. This is one of those conditions that sneak up on you over time. It happens when you have an excessive build up of scar tissue, that – when related to GERD – is thanks to repeated heartburn and acid reflux.

When you have GERD, your acid reflux causes damage to your esophagus lining – and as time progresses, your body builds up layer upon layer of scar tissue. This causes severe restriction in your throat, and swallowing becomes very difficult.

Doctors will treat an esophageal stricture by dilating or stretching your esophagus. This procedure might have to happen more than once, though acid-blocking medication like proton pump inhibitors (PPIs) help prevent its return.

4: Throat and Voice Problems

If you ignore GERD, you may have to deal with additional throat and voice problems. A recurring sore throat is dealt with by visiting an ENT doctor. Once you are there, the ENT specialist will look deep into your larynx with special tools. Often they will see that the little bones that open and close your vocal cords have become swollen. Redness around the vocal cords is typical of acid reflux disease. Common symptoms are a hoarse or raspy voice.

The sphincter at the top of your esophagus is just below your vocal cords, and if this does not work well you'll have cord dysfunction. If digestive juices from the stomach are allowed all the way up into your vocal cord area, they will become irritated. This is called laryngopharyngeal reflux or LPR.

These problems will have a profoundly negative effect on your throat and larynx. You will experience a dry cough, and vocal problems – which becomes challenging for public speakers or singers. If you suffer from GERD and have recurring problems with your throat, then you must go and see a doctor!

5: Breathing Problems

GERD can affect your breathing, and I do not have to tell you how hazardous that can be. When you find it difficult to catch your breath, it will affect every facet of your life. GERD can lead to recurrent pneumonia, and in this case, reflux symptoms must be treated with surgery as soon as possible.

You need to be careful when pneumonia is related to acid reflux. The medications that are used to treat GERD, can make the pneumonia worse, thanks to the various bacteria that causes the condition. They are very hard to treat. That's why I say that pneumonia that continues to recur along with reflux is best treated with surgery, as medication can aggravate your condition.

Both asthma and pneumonia can become worse because of GERD. Even if you do not have these lung conditions, your breathing can still deteriorate – and you'll get shortness of breath.

These treatments can be very risky, and life threatening. The PPI GERD medication we spoke about before, can greatly increase your risk of getting pneumonia. According to several medical studies, these meds may promote bacteria growth, and they suppress coughing which helps the patient clear their lungs.

Asthma causes severe suffering and can be life threatening. Trying to take a deep breath without success is alarming. Research indicates that 70% of all people that have asthma also suffer from acid reflux. Asthma can be difficult to treat.

Reflux is relatively easy to fix with surgery. So if caustic juices from the stomach are refluxing into the breathing airways and triggering asthma then surgery is indicated and can significantly improve an asthma sufferer's quality of life.

6: Tooth Decay

It is bad enough that your teeth have to struggle with the food you eat – but when stomach acids climb the esophagus and spill into your mouth it will wear away your teeth. You will experience a sour taste in your mouth as the acid washes over your teeth, damaging your tooth enamel.

It's a horrible consequence of acid reflux, and people who live with acid-reflux-induced-erosion, are often completely unaware of the damage that it's done to their teeth, until it is too late!

As time passes, tooth decay sets in as a direct result of GERD, which leads to severe teeth problems. Depending on the severity of your GERD symptoms, your tooth decay can happen after a long time, or quite quickly. If the sour taste in your mouth persists repeatedly, from your stomach acids spilling into your mouth – your back teeth will suffer intense consequences.

7: Chronic Cough

Having a chronic cough is another common side effect of GERD. Acid reflux can cause a persistent cough – but in a few cases, this cough is a direct result of non-acidic stomach contents.

- There are 20 different chronic cough causes
- GERD is the second most common cause, after allergies

- 62% of people with a chronic cough have more than one cause
- 75% of the time, people don't even know they have reflux problems
- Specialist therapy cures 98% of all people
- You'll need a 24-hour PH or impedence study to diagnose a GERD induced associated, bitter or irritating cough

8: Sleep Problems

Sleep disorder is another common problem that affects GERD sufferers. Quality, REM sleep is important for good health and good quality of life. Finding a comfortable position to sleep in, that does not affect acid reflux, heartburn or churning stomach acids is near impossible. A lot of people even find that when they lie down, their slight heartburn becomes worse. GERD makes falling asleep, staying asleep and being comfortable very difficult. As a result, healthy sleep is interrupted and rare.

Did you know that...?

GERD is one of the leading causes of disturbed sleep among people between the ages of 45 and 64. (2002 NSF *Sleep in America* poll)

How GERD interferes with your sleeping patterns:

- Patients are woken up with the pain and discomfort from heartburn, which happens when their stomach acids climb their esophagus and eats away at their esophageal lining.

- When stomach acids climb to the top of the throat or larynx, it can induce a coughing attack, or severe choking.

- Patients wake up when a small amount of stomach acid spills into their mouths, as they regurgitate while sleeping.

- According to medical research, GERD is a risk factor for sleep apnea. This disorder causes the person to stop breathing repeatedly as they sleep. The stomach acid causes their voice box to spasm, which blocks the air passages and prevents air from getting into their lungs.

GERD is not a nice condition to have while trying to sleep. The mere act of sleeping makes GERD more likely. As soon as a patient lies down, the risk of intensified acid reflux is present. This is in contrast to standing or sitting positions, which naturally keep stomach acids in your stomach, because of gravity. Lying on your back or side however, makes stomach acid flow into all the wrong places.

Swallowing is also a problem while sleeping, as you tend to do it less. Your esophagus contracts less, which means it is not forcing anything down, or preventing anything from coming back up. As you sleep, you produce less saliva, which normally plays a key role in returning the PH levels in your esophagus to normal, after acid reflux.

9: Barrett's Esophagus

Barrett's esophagus is when your normal, healthy tissue that lines your esophagus changes to become something that resembles your intestinal lining. In total, around 15% of all patients that suffer from severe GERD will develop Barrett's esophagus.

This condition does not present any specific symptoms or side effects. In fact, GERD symptoms are the same in patients with Barrett's esophagus. The only real difference is that it increases your chance of getting esophageal adenocarcinoma – a very serious, fatal cancer of the esophagus.

People that have Barrett's esophagus do carry a higher risk of developing this cancer. We currently do not know the true incidence of this cancer, but it is estimated that it has increased 800% in recent years and is felt due to reflux.

In the past, if Barrett's was worsening, a person would need there esophagus removed and replaced by some other part of their intestines which never worked as well as the esophagus. It is a big operation with side effects. Now there are some new techniques that can get rid of some forms of Barrett's before it turns to cancer and are done endoscopically. It is called *endoscopic ablation therapy.*

I believe anyone with Barrett's should consider having a laparoscopic Nissen Fundoplication and hopefully avoid the more severe forms of the disease.

10: Esophageal Cancer

Battling Barrett's esophagus is often the reason for the increased risk of this type of cancer. Esophageal cancer is more likely to develop in patients with this condition, but some patients go from inflammation to cancer without developing Barrett's. Inflammation is a common known precursor to cancer.

Right now, GERD is just a hassle in your life. It gives you manageable pain that can be eased with medication. But you must remember that it can easily cause these other health concerns. If you feel like you might have GERD, or you have already been diagnosed – then perhaps it is time to have another chat with your doctor about it. A lot of these conditions can be cured or treated, and you have the power to take these steps now before anything serious occurs. You must initiate the treatment.

Why Is Cancer Of The Esophagus On The Rise?

The bottom line is we don't know. But it does correlate with the rising incidence of reflux disease. I think that the incidence of reflux is skyrocketing because of years of overeating, a combination of medications, and food additives. I think the incidence of adenocarcinoma of the esophagus is skyrocketing because we are not treating the cause.

Esophageal cancer is a devastating disease and when it occurs, it rapidly progresses from symptoms to death, usually in one to two years, if left untreated. Long-term survival is very poor. It is rare to find esophageal cancer before it has spread or metastasized. Once it has spread, survival is around 5%. If you can catch it early, have your esophagus surgically removed, and get chemotherapy your survival can jump to 70%. *So if you are having symptoms, get an endoscopy!*

There is an interesting article written in the Wall Street Journal October 10, 2005 titled: *"The Hidden Dangers of Heartburn"*[1]. Take a few minutes to Google it, so that you can add to your heartburn knowledge. For a more scientific explanation, you may want to read the work of the pathologist from the University of Southern California, Dr. Parakrama Chandrasoma. His book is available on amazon.com.

Some of my beliefs come from these writings.

The esophagus is made up of four different types of cells. The upper two thirds or more of the esophagus has a cell type called squamous. The lower part has three different types of columnar cells. And these lower three types of cells are the ones that when things go haywire, turn to cancer. So here is the interesting part.

The only thing that all the current medications do is reduce acid produced in the stomach. They do not prevent reflux of any of

---

1 Parker-Pope, Tara (2005). *The Wall Street Journal*. The Hidden Dangers of Heartburn.
   http://www.post-gazette.com/pg/05283/586020.stm

the juices into the esophagus or have any influence on the ability of these other juices to damage the lower esophagus. These other juices are bacteria, bile, and digestive enzymes and maybe others. These medications have almost eradicated the severe forms of damage to the squamous type cells, those cells in the upper part of the esophagus. As a result, we are seeing a decrease in squamous cancer of the esophagus, esophagitis, esophageal ulcers, and esophageal strictures.

Esophageal strictures occur when the squamous cells are ulcerated and heal with scar tissue that narrows over time. These medications have no protective influence on the other three cell types and we are *absolutely* seeing an increase in inflammation on these types of cells, despite the widespread availability of acid suppressing medication. In other words, these medications do not reduce inflammation in the cells below the squamous cells, the ones that develop into adenocarcinoma of the esophagus, the cancer that is skyrocketing. Inflammation is a precursor to cancer. In other words, it starts with some form of inflammation caused by some chemical in the refluxed juices.

The inflammation process causes the genetics within the cells to cause these cells to change. When cellular change occurs, sometimes things go wrong and the cells change into cancer cells. Normal cellular growth is a controlled event. Cancer cells grow uncontrolled. *So, how do we prevent normal cells from changing into cancer cells?*

We need to identify the chemical precursor that causes the switch and block it. There are no medications at this time that can do that for the cells that turn into adenocarcinoma. It makes sense that most likely these juices that reflux into the esophagus are the cause and if we block reflux of juices up into the esophagus where they do not belong, then the steps that lead to cancer will not occur.

Surgery has been proven to prevent reflux, when performed by experienced surgeons, in 95% or greater of the time. I think gastro esophageal reflux is a premalignant disease and often needs surgical treatment.

We have a new testing procedure that measures air and any juice that goes up into the esophagus where it does not belong. It is called *impedence esophageal manometry*. It has proven that the medications used for heartburn and other reflux symptoms do not prevent reflux and surgery does.

7 Conditions That Mimic GERD

GERD is a condition all on its own, though like many other conditions, it shares symptoms with other diseases – which can cause a lot of confusion. This is why it is very important to communicate your symptoms to a doctor, so that they can pin point exactly which condition is affecting you.

GERD may seem like an 'easy' condition to manage, but you should not take it lightly. Keep in mind though, that stressing about it is not going to help your symptoms, it will make them worse. So stay calm and get help.

The first step is getting your condition diagnosed correctly. Doing this early will help you treat your condition, and prevent any secondary problems from arising. But part of this process, is understanding that many other problems can mimic the symptoms associated with GERD. Bring these concerns up with your doctor and make sure you are tested. You will be able to narrow it down until a correct diagnosis is found.

In some cases, you might have another condition, and GERD to deal with.

1: Stomach Ulcers and Gastritis

Stomach ulcers are basically sores in the stomach. Gastritis is where the stomach has a sunburned red appearance, which is inflammation. Both can be caused by bacteria called Helicobacter pylori. Some stomach ulcers and gastritis are caused by medications like ibuprofen, naproxen, and aspirin and many others. Bile from further down into the intestine can go backwards into the stomach and cause irritation and gastritis. And sometimes we simply do not know why they occur. However, they both are very treatable with medication and if left untreated can cause bleeding and life threatening problems.

The symptoms are very much like GERD symptoms. Typically, patients report a burning sensation just below their breastbone. The symptoms are always present, but vary in the intensity, or how much it hurts at different times during the day. Eating either worsens or helps the pain.

An endoscopy is required to differentiate GERD from stomach ulcers or gastritis and sometimes people have all three.

2: Heart Disease

Heart disease is a blanket term used to describe any number of heart-related diseases. It is commonly used to describe the potential for a heart attack. GERD and heart disease share many common symptoms. Most often Coronary Heart Disease is confused with the symptoms of GERD – like chest pain, which is actually thought to be a bad case of heartburn.

GERD sufferers also deal with shortness of breath, but this is a big symptom of the more serious Coronary Heart Disease. Anyone with heartburn or chest pain needs a cardiac evaluation if they have other risk factors like family history, diabetes, hypertension, or hypercholesterolemia.

3: Gallbladder Disease

 Some 25 million people have been diagnosed with this disease. The gallbladder is meant to store and concentrate bile. Bile is like green soap and helps digest fat for nutrition. We humans make way too much bile and do not need an organ to store and concentrate bile. The way bile gets in and out of the gallbladder is not a mechanically sound system and it is my belief that we overburden the gallbladder because we make so much bile that inflammation occurs and disease and or stones follow. Whatever the true cause is does not really matter, because when it is diseased it needs to be surgically removed. Fortunately, we function very well without a gallbladder.

The symptoms can mimic GERD and particularly heartburn symptoms. The typical symptom is a pain of discomfort just below the ribs on the right side that come and go at will. When they are gone, they are gone. Then they come back another day. But sometimes it is a burning sensation just below the breastbone in the middle and that mimics GERD.

4: Pleuritis or Costochondritis

Pleuritis is caused by a viral or bacterial infection. But when the infection clears up, so does this condition.

Costochondritis is an inflammation of the cartilage on your ribs, which anchor your breastbone. This inflammation causes pain along the sternum. It is often related to infection or injury in some manner, and is treated with basic anti-inflammatory and pain medications.

As both of these conditions cause swelling on the lungs or ribcage, which leads to shortness of breath – it is mistaken as a bad case of heartburn. The best way to differentiate the symptoms of costochondritis from GERD is by pushing on the breastbone. If it causes more pain with more pressure, most likely it is costochondritis.

Pleuritis is more difficult to diagnose and may require imaging studies on the lungs. In severe cases when there is a lot of pain, people might think that they are experiencing a heart attack. To prevent this confusion and get the right diagnosis and treatment for this issue – you must speak to your doctor. If your dominant symptom is pain in your chest area, it may not be GERD at all. Either way, you definitely need to consult a medical professional to find out.

5: Achalasia

Achalasia is a condition of the nervous system of the esophagus. The nervous system tells the muscles of the esophagus to first squeeze at the top, then the middle, then the lower end and push food through the relaxing sphincter into the stomach. With achalasia, all the muscles squeeze at the same time and the sphincter does not relax. This makes it very hard for food to make it from the tongue to the stomach and hurts.

Every patient that I have ever diagnosed with achalasia came to the office complaining of heartburn and thought they had GERD. However, achalasia patients do not improve with the typical acid reducing medications and all complain of difficulty swallowing both solids and liquids. We diagnose achalasia with esophageal manometry where the squeeze pressures of the muscles of the esophagus are measured. A tiny tube in placed in the esophagus and the patient is asked to swallow small cups of water. Achalasia is treated by surgery, botox, or dilation. But all the treatments only improve symptoms and none actually cures them.

6: *Eosinophilic Esophagitis*

Eosinophilic Esophagitis happens as a result of an allergic reaction. While it is not a disease, it is very dangerous. Mostly reported in children, it has also recently become prolific in adults. This condition and the many similarities it shares with GERD, has resulted in misdiagnosis for a lot of adults. Vomiting, abdominal pain, nausea and trouble swallowing are a few related symptoms. It may cause a narrowing of the esophagus and difficulty swallowing. Patients have typical GERD symptoms. Diagnosis is made by taking biopsies at the time of endoscopy. Treatment is difficult and sometimes involves taking anti-inflammatory steroids.

7: *Functional Heartburn*

This is definitely one of the closest related conditions to GERD. While they are very similar, functional heartburn is slightly different. Medical professionals refer to this condition as 'functional' because a patient can live without ever having to treat their heartburn problem and there is no known tissue damage. We don't know why, but the gut becomes extra sensitive.

As we've seen in this book, leaving a condition untreated is never a good idea. Take note of your symptoms and report them to your doctor. If you undergo a few simple tests, your doctor should be able to determine whether you have functional heartburn or GERD. Treatment can be difficult and often involves taking anti-depressant type medications that decrease gut sensitivity.

Diagnostic Process

The only way you can really find out what ails you is to take part in the diagnostic process. Doctors use diagnostic testing to see how severe your problem is, and if it has caused, or is a result of, any number of alternate surrounding issues. You must have a diagnosis before you can begin treatment of your disease. This is the only way you can take charge, and begin solving your health problems.

Specific tests are available that will help you find out if Gastro esophageal Reflux Disease is something you've developed, or if it's just simple heartburn. When you consult with your doctor, they will determine which tests you should take and why. To give you some more grounding on the diagnosis process, here are the current tests available to you.

The Consultation and EGD

On meeting with your doctor for the first time, you will need to disclose and discuss your medical history. If you've been having digestive and heartburn symptoms for some time – that could be enough motivation to do some testing. Your medical professional will also be interested in your family history, as it can contain clues about which diseases or conditions you are most likely to get. After establishing how prone you are to certain illnesses, your doctor will decide how they are going to go about the diagnostic process.

Endoscopy

Upper gastrointestinal endoscopy or esophagogastroduodenoscopy (EGD) is the most common diagnostic process involved in determining whether you suffer from GERD. When you do an EGD, a tube that contains an optical system must be swallowed. As this tube slides down your throat and into your gastrointestinal tract, esophagus, duodenum and stomach – the doctor will be able to see if any damage has occurred.

Patients that show symptoms of acid reflux do not have anything unusual going on in their esophagus. It can look completely normal. But sometimes in more serious cases, the lining in your esophagus is inflamed and esophagitis is present. If your endoscopy shows superficial breaks in your lining, or deeper breaks there, erosions and ulcers are present. In this case, GERD can be diagnosed with confidence. The great thing about an endoscopy is that it will illuminate which symptoms of GERD you are suffering from – namely Barrett's esophagus, strictures and ulcers. A biopsy can also be performed during this process.

The endoscopy may also reveal if there are other problems that are causing GERD to flare up. Problems like ulcers, cancers of the duodenum and stomach, and general inflammation are observed.

Biopsies

While you can get a biopsy of your esophagus during your endoscopic procedure, they're not considered very effective when diagnosing GERD. On the other hand, they are extremely useful when identifying if certain cancers are present, or if the esophageal inflammation is being caused by something else, like an infection. These biopsies are more commonly used to diagnose Barrett's esophagus, as the cellular changes will be evident.

The latest medical studies also suggest that a biopsy will show wide spaces between cell linings, a clear indication that damage is happening as a result of GERD. This can't be seen by the naked eye.

Barium X-ray

A barium x-ray or barium swallow, are basically x-rays where barium is used to find and identify abnormalities in your digestive tract. It is administered by drinking a chalky liquid that contains colored barium. This liquid then coats the walls of your stomach and esophagus, and will show up on x-rays. Your doctor will then be able to see abnormalities like ulcers, strictures, erosions and hiatal hernias.

Keep in mind that a barium x-ray is not a reliable diagnostic test for GERD, as it isn't sensitive enough. This test is administered when patients have difficulty swallowing or if an overall picture of the shape of the esophagus and its position in the thoracic is needed.

Impedence

An impedence test can only be administered at selected medical centers. Most centers don't have the capability to run this kind of test. Similar to the 24-hour PH test, a tube is inserted through the nose of the patient, and is slid down into the esophagus until it reaches the

LES. The test itself measures the movement of air and liquid from the stomach into the esophagus. This test can be very valuable for people suffering from bile reflux symptoms – because they get normal results from a 24-hour PH probe. During the 24-hour impedence measurement, a 24-hour PH probe reading can also be taken. Impedence testing can't be done with the same PH measuring device that is currently clipped to your esophageal lining. It is by far the best test for patients with asthma, chronic cough, or a variable response to acid reducing mediations.

Manometry

To perform a manometry test, a small tube is passed through the nose until it reaches the esophagus. Before the procedure begins, the nose and throat of the patient are numbed. When the tube is in place, the patient must swallow. The pressure readings from your esophageal muscle contractions are then measured, to determine the motility of your esophageal function. You can also test your LES muscle pressure at the same time. These tests help doctors determine whether there is an issue with the strength of your esophageal contractions. While the test won't confirm that symptoms of GERD are present, it will inform the doctor if esophageal motility problems are a contributing factor to the disease. Almost all patients that describe difficulty swallowing food need this test.

PH Testing

A 24-hour esophageal PH test is done to determine the amount of time that acid remains in the esophagus. PH is just a fancy name for acidity. A tiny tube is inserted into the nose and is slid down into the esophagus. On the very tip of this tube is a sensor that responds to acid. At the other end of the tube is the recording device on the outside of the patient's body. Every time stomach acids are forced back up into the esophagus, the sensor is stimulated and it records the reflux episode. After 24 hours, the tube comes out, and the doctor can then analyze the recorded refluxes.

This is a very reliable test for acid reflux. I find it most useful if a patient does not have typical reflux symptoms or does not respond to acid reducing medication adequately. It will prove whether they have acid reflux or not. It cannot prove whether they have non-acid reflux, and for that, we need impedence testing. For example, a patient may primarily complain of chest pain, and the medications seem to help, but do not resolve the symptoms. They get a normal cardiac evaluation. Then we do endoscopy and everything looks pretty normal. This patient would be an excellent candidate for 24 hour PH testing.

Common Problems Resulting From GERD Medication

After the diagnostic process is complete, and you've established that you have GERD, it's time to look at treatment options. Most patients will require a basic prescription medication, but for a select few who have severe symptoms, surgery may be the only option. Patients that are on prescribed medication have many options available to them.

Did you know that...?

Some medications taken for other medical conditions can trigger GERD symptoms

The type of medication that is prescribed will depend on the intensity of your symptoms, and a few surrounding factors – like allergies. After speaking with your doctor, you'll decide on which medicines you'd like to test out. You must be aware that every medication causes a reaction in your body. If you react negatively to your medication, stop taking it. All prescription medication have side effects, so keep a look out for them when you start your course.

Prilosec

Prilosec comes in a delayed release capsule, and is ingested orally. Here are a few of the milder side effects:

- Nausea
- Abdominal pains
- Vomiting
- Headaches
- Gas
- Diarrhea

Allergic reactions can happen, along with side effects that are more significant. If you experience any of these, seek immediate medical assistance.

- Difficulty breathing
- Hives
- Throat or tongue swelling
- Face swelling

Nexium

Another medication that is administered orally in delayed release capsule form. There are several side effects to look out for, and if you experience any of them consult with your doctor as soon as you can. This is especially true if these side effects persist for quite a while.

- Nausea
- Stomach pain
- Drowsiness
- Constipation
- Diarrhea

- Headaches
- Dry mouth

If you experience an allergic or more severe reaction, you need to report these to your doctor immediately, or seek medical help.

- Weakness
- Hives or rashes
- Hoarseness
- Yellow eyes or skin
- Bleeding or bruising
- Difficulty breathing
- Face, tongue and mouth swelling
- Chills and fever

These are not the only indicators that you are having an allergic reaction, so remember to speak to your doctor about what else you need to focus on.

Prevacid

Prevacid is another type of delayed release capsule medication. Taken orally, these are the different potential side effects that you need to look out for:

- Abdominal pains
- Nausea
- Headaches
- Constipation
- Diarrhea

Just like the other medication, this one also has more severe effects and allergic reactions. Do not forget to discuss all of the medications that you are allergic to, with your doctor before he prescribes your GERD medication. It will lower your chance of having a reaction.

Aciphex

Many patients find that this medication is tolerated well, and it is a popular option. There are only two main common side effects of this medication, diarrhea and getting headaches. This does not mean there aren't other side effects, but these are usually caused by a severe allergic reaction. Please look out for these, and inform your doctor as soon as they manifest:

- Bleeding or bruising
- Sore throat, chills and fever
- Irregular heartbeat
- Hives or rashes
- Chest or bone pain
- Face or mouth swelling
- Abdominal pains
- Difficulty breathing

This is not the complete list of side effects, so please ask your doctor to inform you about any others of concern.

Dexilant

Though GERD medications often cause nausea, gas and diarrhea – you also need to look out for upper respiratory tract infections! This is a very real side effect. Bad allergic reactions to Dexilant will include these symptoms:

- Seizure

- Fainting
- Depression
- Facial swelling
- Hives, rashes and itching
- Difficulty breathing or chest tightness
- Pain in the calves or bones

As always, you should speak with your doctor about the additional side effects that this medication could cause, especially when associated with allergic reactions.

Tagamet

Another popular medication for GERD, Tagamet's most common side effect is diarrhea. However, you should also look out for:

- Drowsiness
- Headache
- Dizziness

Along with the many other common allergic side effects from the other medications on the market, you need to monitor yourself for these as well:

- Muscle and joint pain
- Hair loss
- Breast enlargement or lumps
- Sexual difficulty
- Depression, confusion, agitation and anxiety

Pepcid

Among the potential side effects of both Pepcid and Pepcid AC are:

- Constipation
- Diarrhea
- Headache
- Dizziness

Make sure that if you experience any of these allergic reactions, you immediately consult your doctor. Having one or more of these are very serious side effects. Keep an eye out for:

- Seizure
- Face swelling
- Difficulty breathing
- Hives, rashes and itching
- Irregular heartbeat
- Chest tightness

Gaviscon

Gaviscon, another widely used GERD medication, has some of the least potential side effects of all the medications. The two main side effects are constipation and diarrhea. Along with the 'common' symptoms that surface from severe allergic reactions – you also need to be careful of slow reflexes, muscle weakness and loss of appetite.

Gaviscon makes a wafer of thick material that when in the upright position sits on top of your food and makes it difficult for the stomach juices to reflux into the esophagus.

The general rule with all medication is that if you experience a change in your body or behavior after using the prescription, then you need to speak to your doctor.

Surgery...What Are Your Options?

Reflux is a mechanical problem, not a chemistry problem. The medications used to treat heartburn and reflux related symptoms change the chemistry inside the stomach, but do not prevent reflux. We have proven this with a test called **esophageal impedence manometry**. The test measures air and liquids that reflux into the esophagus from the stomach. People on medication for heartburn and reflux related symptoms still experience reflux. Surgery is the only known way to prevent reflux.

The problem is a broken one-way valve, and much like the valve on a toilet, it will leak until fixed. You do not have to rush out and fix it, but the toilet will waste water until you do and you will have to live with that irritating leaky noise.

There are several components to the functioning one-way valve or more scientifically the so-called lower esophageal sphincter. All or some of the components may be broken. For this valve to function properly, it needs a certain shape and it needs to be within the abdominal cavity, not the thoracic cavity where the lungs and heart are located.

A muscle called the diaphragm separates the thoracic and abdominal cavities. The esophagus travels from the tongue through this muscle to reach the abdominal cavity and extends a few centimeters into the abdominal cavity. The muscles within the wall of the esophagus and the muscles within the wall of the stomach are different. They are oriented in different directions. The orientation of these muscles gives the valve a particular shape. The shape has a sling–like look to it. Take your index finger and place it on your gums just above your front teeth. Now pucker your lips tightly around your finger. Your lip should protrude out onto your finger for a few centimeters. That is what the lower esophageal sphincter should look like. If your lip only slightly protrudes onto your finger, say less than a centimeter, then it would leak.

You can have reflux with or without a hiatal hernia. A hiatal hernia is present when all or part of the sphincter is above the diaphragm where the heart and lungs are, the thoracic cavity. Basically, the support structures around the sphincter area weaken. The pressures in the abdominal cavity are positive and the pressures in the thoracic cavity are negative. This difference in pressure causes the sphincter and sometimes the stomach to protrude into the thoracic cavity.

The positive pressure pushes it into the thoracic cavity and the negative pressure pulls it into the thoracic cavity. The end result - the valve loses its proper shape and is in the wrong cavity to function as a one-way valve. If a hiatal hernia is present, the hernia will need to be repaired for the valve to function properly and for the re-built valve to have proper shape.

There have been a myriad of methods to surgically treat reflux, but I am going to only spend time talking about the three that I feel are most valid for today, the Nissen fundoplication, transoral incisionless fundoplication (TIF), and the Stretta procedure..

First off, let's get a few terms out of the way. Fundus means ear shape. The upper left hand side of the stomach has an ear shape to it, and we call it the fundus.

Plication is just a fancy word for suturing something together. So a fundoplication implies we suture the fundus into a certain position.

Rudolph Nissen began performing this operation in 1955, and the Nissen fundoplication appropriately bears his name. It is not a Nissan, like the car. The fundoplication is the part of the operation where the valve is re-shaped to a shape like your lips puckered around your finger.

Nissen Fundoplication

If you have a hiatal hernia and reflux, you need both a hiatal hernia repair and the valve reshaped. The Nissen fundoplication is a two-step operation.

- Step one is bringing the esophagus back down into the abdominal cavity and repair the weakened support structures of the diaphragm.
- Step two is the fundoplication where the valve is reshaped by taking the fundus of the stomach and wrapping it around the lower part of the esophagus, which now resides a few centimeters into the abdominal cavity.

The overall result is that *puckered lip* look within the abdominal cavity.

The operation is done through tiny incisions called laparoscopy. I have done the procedure since 1992 and as an outpatient procedure for 15 years. The operation takes me about one hour to complete, and patients are usually headed home after about one hour of recovery. It does hurt, but the pain is well tolerated with liquid pain medicine taken orally.

Patients can do everything within one week, and most patients can do most things within a few days, much like gallbladder surgery. Compared to other surgeries, it is a very low risk operation. There is a period of time when patients have difficulty swallowing food. So they start with mashed potatoes and move to soft, moist, chewable food, and later regular food. Most people can eat a few foods such as an enchilada within the first week, but steak, bread and gummy rice may take a while and it varies person to person. I personally have never had a patient where this difficulty swallowing did not return to normal. There are, however, published reports from other surgeons where this difficulty swallowing never resolved. We call difficulty swallowing – *dysphagia*.

Patients can stop their medications for reflux the night of surgery. Patients wake up from anesthesia with the feeling that the reflux problem is gone.

Did you know that…?
Reflux surgery is safe and
with a 95% success rate.

There is this thing called *gas bloat* that does occur. I think it is related to swallowing air and a problem with the stomach not emptying its contents into the rest of the gastrointestinal tract properly. It does tend to go away. I personally have had no patient come to my office complaining of this long-term and no patient who did not recommend the operation to others because of gas bloat. If you swallow air, it will go rapidly from the mouth to the anus, and you will fart. Usually the passed gas does not have an odor because it is just swallowed air. Over time, most people learn to not swallow air so much.

TIF or Transoral Incisionless Fundoplication

That means a large scope and instrument is passed from the mouth, through the esophagus, and down into the stomach. Once in the stomach a hook-like wire pulls the sphincter into a proper shape and then the instrument sutures or plicates it into this position. Because it is done through the mouth, there are no incisions.

The pain following the procedure is on the same magnitude of the Nissen fundoplication and the same liquid pain medicine taken by mouth is used. Patients are instructed to stay on a liquid or extremely soft diet for about a mouth. It is important for patients to not vomit or retch, or the sutures might tear out and the valve may lose its renewed shape and it may cause a tear in the esophagus. Most patients spend one night in the hospital and are doing most things within a week.

In general, I believe a surgeon should do the least surgery to accomplish the goal. So I believe in this procedure for patients that do not need a hiatal hernia repair.

There are some reports that have followed patients for three years after surgery and the results are similar to the Nissen fundoplication. Some reports suggest there is less gas bloat, but they need a larger study group to prove this is true.

However, I have been doing the Nissen fundoplication for many years and do not see significant gas bloat that does not resolve.

Both operations re-build the one-way valve and reflux resolves. Patients often realize as soon as they fully awaken from anesthesia that the reflux feeling is gone. The medications for reflux are stopped the day of surgery.

The TIF procedure does not repair hiatal hernias. Hiatal hernia repair is a standard part of the Nissen fundoplication, but not possible with the TIF procedure. Most people with reflux have a significant hiatal hernia and in my opinion are not candidates for the TIF. The sutures that are placed with the device are not as secure as with the sutures we use in the Nissen procedure and in my opinion the procedure is not as durable.

In other words, if you retch and vomit after the Nissen procedure it is unlikely that you will disrupt the repair. If you retch soon after the TIF procedure there is a high risk of disrupting the repair. Patients are asked to be on a liquid diet for one month and most patients find that difficult. So when a patient has reflux and no significant hiatal hernia, then I give them the option of TIF or Nissen. Most choose the Nissen procedure because of my 22 plus years experience with the procedure, the early post op durability of the procedure, the fact that they do not want to be on a liquid diet for a month, and it requires an over night hospitalization.

Stretta Procedure

The Stretta is a procedure that came and went and is now available again. It works for the right patient. Like the TIF procedure, it does not fix hiatal hernias. So if a patient has reflux and no hiatal hernia then this might be a procedure for them. It strengthens a weak one-way valve by using radiofrequency heat to cause tiny little burns into the muscle. The healing process causes the muscle to become stronger. It is done by an endoscope through the mouth and requires no abdominal incisions. It takes about an hour. Patients go home the same day as the procedure. It hurts for a few days and the pain is easily controlled with pain medicine. The procedure disappeared for several years because the company had financial issues that arose from the fact that insurance companies would rarely approve the procedure. Now even Medicare approves it. About 60 million people in the USA have reflux. In my opinion about 25% of those do not have a hiatal hernia and may be a candidate.

Living Without GERD: Choosing a Life You Love

It's an unfortunate diagnosis, but sometimes medication simply isn't enough for people that suffer from severe GERD. Sometimes patients try all of the medications one by one, and yet side effects persist with all of the prescriptions. A consultation with your doctor may reveal that surgery is actually the right path for you to take, based on your individual diagnosis and reactions. Whatever the path – either medication or surgery – the end result needs to be the same. The complete alleviation or elimination of GERD.

Now that you've been treating your GERD, all you have to do is keep following up on your care, by taking your prescription meds and changing your diet if that's what must happen. You must monitor your own health, and be wary of returning symptoms associated with acid reflux and GERD. At the end of the day, you need to take care of yourself to prevent the symptoms of GERD from ever coming back into your life.

The Good News!

There is some good news once you've had surgery, or have stuck to a medication schedule. Your quality of life will significantly improve! GERD can be a horrible disease that disrupts every part of your life, from morning to evening. Many are so badly affected, that it becomes impossible to take part in family or social situations, where food is present. Now that you have treated your GERD, you will begin to experience many nice benefits on a daily basis.

First of all, sleep will be a lot more comfortable. You will not have to spend all night tossing and turning, in pain, because lying down causes your acid reflux to flare up. You'll be able to sleep through the entire night, without waking up. No more GERD symptoms waking you up at night! It will improve your ability to fall asleep and the quality of the sleep that you get. This alone will change your life.

Great Possibilities

Wouldn't it be amazing to enjoy a full meal, without having to worry about that terrible burning in your chest afterwards? Once again, you will be able to experience meal times with family and friends, pain free and full of life. That's what your future can be when you get rid of your GERD symptoms. But eating isn't the only activity that you'll be able to enjoy again! You will be able to do things that you have not done in ages.

Your sex life will once again become an exciting and appealing prospect. GERD causes painful burning, which makes bending and any intimacy extremely difficult. But you can regain this portion of your life. You do not have to resign yourself to the fact that sex will never be enjoyable again!

Final Words

Regain Your Freedom

Once your GERD is treated, you can seize control of your life. Your symptoms will not dictate what you can do anymore – it will not interfere with your life. Just imagine the better quality of life you'll have when GERD isn't a constant worry. And wouldn't it be incredible to never have to take any medication ever again? No more dependency on prescription drugs!

There are so many benefits, including never having to wake up choking or coughing again. Right now, you live your life around your GERD symptoms. It affects your eating and sleeping habits, your sex life and dictates how active you get to be. What you need is a carefree life, where burning pain does not interrupt your day. Remember all the things you could do when you were GERD free? You can be that again!

GERD is a disease that should not be ignored, overlooked or self-treated. Heartburn may be common, but it is also an indicator that you have GERD. Do not underestimate, dismiss or suffer unnecessarily with heartburn.

GERD is a very real problem. Obvious symptoms may lead you to a diagnosis, but there are less obvious symptoms that you need to be aware of as well. If you continue to ignore these red flags, it will lead to future health problems. Most people only have a mild form of GERD that can be controlled with medication and proper diet.

If you think that you might suffer from GERD, you need to contact a doctor right away. Get an accurate diagnosis. GERD is a treatable disease; you do not have to live with it! Work together with your doctor to implement the best treatment plan, and take back your life.

Be healthy, be GERD free!

-Dr. Cliff Thomas

About the Author

Cliff Thomas' life in the medical field began early. His father was a hospital administrator and his uncle was the Chief of Staff and primary physician, so essentially he grew up in a hospital. At 10, he began working in the maintenance department, which evolved into many different jobs around the hospital.

At an early age, Cliff recognized the passion his uncle had for being a doctor. He witnessed it over and over and noticed how his patients responded. That is when the seed was planted. As the years went on, jobs ranged from janitorial to x-ray, to the laboratory and finally to surgery. Cliff realized the best job in the hospital was that of the surgeons'.

He graduated from the University of Texas at Austin in 1979, finishing medical school at the University of Texas Medical Branch in 1984. He then went on to complete a 5-year General Surgery residency and subsequently became an Assistant Professor of Surgery.

His emphasis throughout residency was GI surgery and included extensive experience with the Vertical Banded Gastroplasty for weight loss – a procedure that was later found to have a 70% failure rate.

Cliff then began a hand surgery fellowship but it wasn't long before he realized his real passion was GI surgery. He began his solo general surgery practice in Nacogdoches Texas in 1990, where he continues to have a satellite office today. He chose Nacogdoches because after his experiences with hand surgery in Oakland California, he thought smaller was better.

Cliff became a fellow in the American College of Surgeons (FACS) and was Board Certified by the American Board of Surgery in 1990. 1990 also marked the beginning of laparoscopic surgery, and he quickly found that his skill set fit laparoscopic GI surgery. His advanced laparoscopic experience began in 1992, performing hiatal hernia repairs (Nissen Fundoplications).

At that time, there were only a handful of surgeons in the world performing this procedure. It continues to be a rewarding part of his practice and has many similarities with bariatric surgery.

By the late 1990's Laparoscopic Gastric Bypass was being performed by several surgeons in the United States. Cliff launched his bariatric surgery practice in 2000, after training with some of the most experienced surgeons in the country and doing a mini-fellowship at Parkland in Dallas.

Since then bariatric surgery has become a major part of his practice. In November 2002, he began also performing the Laparoscopic Adjustable Gastric Band and later added the Laparoscopic Sleeve Gastrectomy.

It became clear that Nacogdoches could not support an active bariatric practice, so in 2005 Cliff began practicing in Houston. In that time, Dr. Yusem Nowzaradan and Cliff Thomas performed the largest gastric bypass and gastric sleeve in the world.

Cliff has a passion for what he does, and wakes every morning eager to do more. He gets to use his skillset in surgery and then see and feel how that changes people's lives for the better.